Copyright ©2020 ARNOLD KUNTZ PH.D

CONTENTS

DO CLEANSES WORK?

Proponents of kidney cleansing say that certain foods, beverages, and diets can detoxify the kidneys and body. However, there is currently little scientific research to support these claims.

The National Center for Complementary and Integrative Health (NCCIH) state that there isn't any convincing evidence that detox or cleansing programs actually remove toxins from your body or improve your health. Most people can keep their kidneys healthy by staying hydrated and eating a balanced, healthful diet. However, some herbs and foods that are popular in kidney cleansing programs may have properties that help promote kidney health.

HOW TO CLEANSE THE KIDNEYS

Cleansing the kidneys may aid the removal of toxins from the body. The following tips may help improve kidney health and reduce the risk of kidney disease:

Drink more water

Drinking enough fluid every day is essential to a person's overall health. Water is crucial for digesting food, absorbing nutrients, getting rid of waste and toxins, keeping the skin healthy, and performing a wide range of other bodily functions. Consuming enough water can also help prevent kidney problems, such as kidney stones. According to the National Institute of Diabetes and Digestive and Kidney Diseases (NIDDK), many healthcare professionals recommend drinking six to eight 8-ounce (OZ) glasses of water a day.

Reduce sodium intake

The body needs salt, or sodium, but consuming too much can raise blood pressure, which can increase a person's risk of kidney failure, heart disease, and stroke. The NIDDK recommend that people limit their sodium consumption to less than 2,300 milligrams a day to reduce the risk of chronic kidney disease. People can reduce their sodium intake by eating fewer processed foods and choosing low-sodium or sodium-free options.

Make dietary changes

People can make some simple dietary changes to improve both their kidney health and general health, but it is important to note that the following lists are not for people with preexisting kidney disease.

Consider limiting or avoiding the following foods and beverages:

- Processed foods

- Refined carbohydrates

- Sugar and artificial sweeteners

- Animal proteins, such as beef, pork, and organ meat

- High-sodium foods

- Alcohol

- Caffeine

A person can also try adding these kidney-friendly foods to their diet:

- Berries

- Citrus fruits, such as lemons, limes, and oranges

- Apples

- Low-fat dairy products

- Vegetables

- Whole grains, such as barley, brown rice, and oatmeal

- Lean meats, including chicken and seafood

AN EXAMPLE 2-DAY KIDNEY CLEANSE PLAN

A person should consult a doctor before starting a kidney cleanse or detox regimen, particularly if they have kidney stones or kidney disease. Limiting the duration of cleansing programs to a few days can help reduce the risk of adverse health effects. People who do not have kidney problems may wish to try the following 2-day kidney cleanse plan:

Day 1

A tofu salad is a typical meal to help cleanse the kidneys.

On the first day of cleansing, people can prepare the following three meals:

Morning

Start the day with an 8-oz glass of warm water containing 1 tablespoon (tbsp.) of fresh lemon juice.

Breakfast

For breakfast, blend the following ingredients to make a 12-oz smoothie:

  1 beetroot

half a cucumber

2 apples

the juice of half a lemon

1 inch (in) grated ginger

Lunch

Eat a large, mixed green salad containing:

Grilled chicken or tofu

Half a red onion

1 cup chopped apple

One-quarter cup grapes

Top the salad with sliced almonds. For the dressing, combine:

One-third cup low-fat Greek yogurt

1 tbsp. Dijon mustard

1 teaspoon (tsp.) lemon juice

Salt and pepper to taste

Dinner

For dinner, make an 8-oz smoothie containing:

1 cup coconut water

1 cup blueberries

One-half cup mango

1 cup kale

1 tbsp. lemon juice

1 tbsp. ground flaxseed

Day 2

On the second day, people can eat a more substantial lunch and dinner:

Morning

Start the morning with a cup of green tea containing 1 tbsp. of fresh lemon juice.

Breakfast

Blend the following ingredients to make an 8-oz smoothie:

- 1 cup almond milk

- One-half cup spinach

- One-quarter cup mixed berries

- 1 frozen banana

- 1 tbsp. ground flaxseed

Lunch

Combine the following ingredients and then saute together in olive oil:

- 1 cup cooked brown rice

- One-half cup cooked beans

- One-quarter cup green beans

- One-quarter cup chopped carrots

- 1–2 tsp. minced garlic

Dinner

Make a vegetable soup using the following ingredients:

- 1 sweet potato

- 1 cup carrots

2 celery stalks

1 yellow onion

1 cup tomato

1 can kidney beans

One-quarter cup parsley

2 tsp. minced garlic

4 cups low-sodium vegetable broth

Begin by heating the vegetable broth over medium heat. Chop all of the vegetables and add them to the broth. After cooking the vegetables completely, stir in parsley. Add salt and pepper according to taste.

RISKS AND CONSIDERATIONS

Drinking too much can cause low sodium levels.
Kidney cleanse programs generally encourage people to consume more healthful foods, such as fruits and vegetables. However, although proponents of kidney cleanses say that they offer many health benefits, there is little scientific research to support these claims.

According to the NCCIH, the Food and Drug Administration (FDA) have taken action against several companies offering detox and cleansing products because they made false therapeutic claims about their products or the products contained illegal and potentially harmful ingredients.

For example, the FDA filed a warning letter in 2018 to Ozark Country Herbs, a company that produce a range of herbal products that promise to treat everything from depression and migraine to flu and kidney stones. Although drinking enough water is essential for health, too much fluid can reduce mineral concentrations in the body and lead to health complications. A 2018 case study, for instance, reports that a 67-year-old man developed severe hypernatremia, or low sodium levels in the blood, while performing a kidney cleanse. Hypernatremia is a serious medical condition that can lead to potentially life-threating complications, such as swelling of the brain.

Many kidney cleanses and detox programs also require a person to fast or severely restrict their calorie intake, which can lead to headaches, fatigue, and nutritional imbalances. People who wish to try a kidney cleanse should consult a doctor first and ensure that they are consuming enough calories and electrolytes to support their metabolism.

DOING A NATURAL KIDNEY CLEANSE AT HOME

-Hydration

-Foods

-Teas

-Supplements

-Sample cleanse

-Takeaway

The kidneys are two small organs located on either side of the spine, below the ribs. They play an important role in getting rid of excess waste, balancing electrolytes, and creating hormones. In the absence of disease, a well-rounded diet and adequate water intake are usually enough to keep your kidneys healthy. However, certain foods, herbs, and supplements can help support strong kidneys.

From your morning glass of water to that extra cup of herbal tea, here are four ways to cleanse your kidneys and keep them functioning strong.

1. HYDRATION IS KEY

The adult human body is composed of almost 60 percent water. Every single organ, from the brain to the liver, requires water to function. As the filtration system of the body, the kidneys require water to secrete urine. Urine is the primary waste product that allows the body to get rid of unwanted or unnecessary substances. When water intake is low, urine volume is low. A low urine output may lead to kidney dysfunction, such as the creation of kidney stones. It's crucial to drink enough water so that the kidneys can properly flush out any excess waste materials. This is especially important during a kidney cleanse. The recommended daily intake of fluids is roughly 3.7 liters and 2.7 liters a day for men and women, respectively, according to the Institute of Medicine.

2. CHOOSE FOODS THAT SUPPORT KIDNEY HEALTH

Grapes

Grapes, peanuts, and some berries contain a beneficial plant compound called resveratrol. In one animal study, researchers found that treatment with resveratrol was able to lower kidney inflammation in rats with polycystic kidney disease. A handful of red grapes makes a great afternoon snack and they taste even better frozen.

Cranberries

Cranberries have often been praised for their bladder health benefits. A clinical trial in Nutrition Journal demonstrated that women who consumed sweetened, dried cranberries daily for two weeks experienced a decrease in the incidence of urinary tract infections. Dried cranberries are a deliciously sweet addition to trail mix, salads, or even oatmeal.

Fruit juices

Lemon, orange, and melon juice all contain citric acid, or citrate. Citrate helps prevent kidney stone formation by binding with calcium in urine. This inhibits the growth of calcium crystals, which can lead to kidney stones. In addition, drinking a cup of fresh juice per day can contribute to your daily recommended fluid intake.

Seaweed

Brown seaweed has been studied for its beneficial effects on the pancreas, kidneys, and liver. In a 2014 animal trial, rats fed edible seaweed for a period of 22 days showed a reduction in both kidney and liver damage from diabetes. Try a packet of dried, seasoned seaweed the next time you're craving a crunchy snack.

Calcium-rich foods

Many people believe that avoiding calcium can help to prevent kidney stones. In fact, the opposite is true. Too much urinary oxalate can lead to kidney stones. Calcium is needed to bind with oxalate to reduce the absorption and excretion of this substance. You can meet the recommended daily intake of 1.2 grams of calcium by consuming high-calcium foods, such as soy or almond milk, tofu, and fortified cereals.

3. DRINK KIDNEY-CLEANSING TEAS

Stinging nettle

Stinging nettle is a perennial plant that has long been used in traditional herbal medicine. Stinging nettle leaf contains beneficial compounds that can help to reduce inflammation. It's also high in antioxidants, which help to protect the body and organs from oxidative stress.

Hydrangea

Hydrangea is a gorgeous flowering shrub, well-known for its lavender, pink, blue, and white flowers. A recent animal study found that extracts of Hydrangea paniculate given for three days offered a protective effect against kidney damage. This is likely due to the antioxidant capabilities of the plant.

Sambong

Sambong is a tropical climate shrub, common to countries such as the Philippines and India.

In one study, researchers found that a Blumea balsamifera extract added to calcium oxalate crystals decreased the size of the crystals. This could potentially prevent the formation of kidney stones.

4. SUPPLEMENT WITH SUPPORTIVE NUTRIENTS

Vitamin B-6

Vitamin B-6 is an important cofactor in many metabolic reactions. B-6 is required for the metabolism of glyoxylate, which can become oxalate instead of glycine if B-6 is deficient. As mentioned above, too much oxalate may lead to kidney stones. Supplement with a daily B-complex vitamin that provides at least 50 milligrams of B-6.

Omega-3s

The standard American diet is often high in inflammatory omega-6 fatty acids and low in beneficial omega-3 fatty acids. Research suggests that high levels of omega-6 fatty acids may lead to kidney stone formation. An increase in omega-3s can naturally decrease the metabolism of omega- 6s, with the best intake ratio being 1:1.Supplement with a daily high-quality fish oil containing 1.2 g of both EPA and DHA.

Potassium citrate

Potassium is a necessary element of electrolyte balance and pH balance of urine. Therapy with potassium citrate can potentially help to reduce the formation of kidney stones, especially in people who experience recurring episodes. For those with a history of other kidney problems, talk to your doctor before you take potassium supplements with a daily multivitamin or multimineral that contains potassium.

SAMPLE TWO-DAY KIDNEY CLEANSE

Once you've incorporated these foods, herbs, and supplements into your diet, you may want to consider taking your kidney support to the next level. This sample two-day kidney cleanse is thought to help strengthen your kidneys and detoxify your body, but there's no research to support a cleansing action. This plan, however, utilizes foods to support kidney health.

Day 1

Breakfast: 8 ounces each fresh lemon, ginger, and beet juice, plus 1/4 cup sweetened, dried cranberries

Lunch: Smoothie of 1 cup almond milk, 1/2 cup tofu, 1/2 cup spinach, 1/4 cup berries, 1/2 apple, and 2 tablespoons pumpkin seeds

Dinner: Large mixed-greens salad with 4 ounces lean protein (chicken, fish, or tofu), topped with 1/2 cup grapes and 1/4 cup peanuts

Day 2

Breakfast: Smoothie of 1 cup soy milk, 1 frozen banana, 1/2 cup spinach, 1/2 cup blueberries, and 1 teaspoon spirulina.

Lunch: 1 cup hot millet topped with 1 cup fresh fruit and 2 tablespoons pumpkin seeds

Dinner: Large mixed-greens salad with 4 ounces lean protein (chicken, fish, or tofu), topped with 1/2 cup cooked barley and a drizzle of fresh lemon juice plus 4 ounces each unsweetened cherry juice and orange juice

LIVER

This powerful organ cleans the blood and transforms harmful chemicals for eventual excretion. It reigns over all toxins of the body by cleaning and filtering every ounce of blood and metabolizing all chemical substances, even the good kinds. Bitter foods and foods that promote the body's production of internal antioxidants, especially glutathione, are best for liver detoxification.

Foods that support liver detoxification include:
- Cabbage

- Broccoli

- Garlic

- Beets

- Salad greens

- Lemon juice

- Green apples

Bitter herbs that support liver detoxification include:
- Dandelion

- Yellow dock

KIDNEYS

The role of your two kidneys is to flush waste and toxins from your blood by turning it into urine after it's cleaned by the liver. The kidneys flush water-soluble waste in response to water and electrolyte concentrations.

To support detoxification, drink at least 2 quarts of water daily. You can also consume greens, herbs, and teas, which are weak diuretics that promote kidney detox without throwing your electrolytes out of balance. Some foods flush the kidneys and promote healthy blood pressure, and others act as renal tonics to flush extra toxins and prevent bacteria buildup.

10 SIGNS YOU MAY HAVE KIDNEY DISEASE

1. You're more tired, have less energy or are having trouble concentrating. A severe decrease in kidney function can lead to a buildup of toxins and impurities in the blood. This can cause people to feel tired, weak and can make it hard to concentrate. Another complication of kidney disease is anemia, which can cause weakness and fatigue.

2. You're having trouble sleeping. When the kidneys aren't filtering properly, toxins stay in the blood rather than leaving the body through the urine. This can make it difficult to sleep. There is also a link between obesity and chronic kidney disease, and sleep apnea is more common in those with chronic kidney disease, compared with the general population.

3. You have dry and itchy skin. Healthy kidneys do many important jobs. They remove wastes and extra fluid from your body, help make red blood cells, help keep bones strong and work to maintain the right amount of minerals in your blood. Dry and itchy skin can be a sign of the mineral and bone disease that often accompanies advanced kidney disease, when the kidneys are no longer able to keep the right balance of minerals and nutrients in

your blood.

4. You feel the need to urinate more often. If you feel the need to urinate more often, especially at night, this can be a sign of kidney disease. When the kidneys filters are damaged, it can cause an increase in the urge to urinate. Sometimes this can also be a sign of a urinary infection or enlarged prostate in men.

5. You see blood in your urine. Healthy kidneys typically keep the blood cells in the body when filtering wastes from the blood to create urine, but when the kidney's filters have been damaged, these blood cells can start to "leak" out into the urine. In addition to signaling kidney disease, blood in the urine can be indicative of tumors, kidney stones or an infection.

6. Your urine is foamy. Excessive bubbles in the urine – especially those that require you to flush several times before they go away—indicate protein in the urine. This foam may look like the foam you see when scrambling eggs, as the common protein found in urine, albumin, is the same protein that is found in eggs.

7. You're experiencing persistent puffiness around your eyes. Protein in the urine is an early sign that the kidneys' filters have been damaged, allowing protein to leak into the urine. This puffiness around your eyes can be due to the fact that your kidneys are leaking a large amount of protein in the urine, rather than keeping it in the body.

8. Your ankles and feet are swollen. Decreased kidney function can lead to sodium retention, causing swelling in your feet and ankles. Swelling in the lower extremities can also be a sign of heart disease, liver disease and chronic leg vein problems.

9.   You have a poor appetite. This is a very general symptom, but a buildup of toxins resulting from reduced kidney function can be one of the causes.

10.   Your muscles are cramping. Electrolyte imbalances can result from impaired kidney function. For example, low calcium levels and poorly controlled phosphorus may contribute to muscle cramping.

Foods that support kidney flush:
  -Water

  -Parsley

  -Cilantro

  -Green tea

  -Nettle Alfalfa

Renal tonic foods:
  -Cranberry

  -Juniper berry

GUIDE TO DETOXING KIDNEYS AND LIVER IN A HEALTHY WAY

Detoxing kidneys and liver regularly is essential for maintaining your health because these organs are your natural 'filters'. This means that they suffer the worst of the damage that comes from toxins, which get inside your body. As the environmental pollution stands now, no one can lead a 100% toxin-free life now, so your natural defenses need all the help they can get.

The trick is that detoxing kidneys and liver the wrong way can be harmful to you. Unbalanced diets and some untested 'natural remedies' are a danger in themselves. Therefore, it's imperative you follow a healthy and sound detoxification guide.

WHAT IS A LIVER DETOX?

In order to rid your body of toxins that can build up in your tissues, fat, joints, and brain, your body must excrete them through the complex filtration system of your kidneys and liver. A liver detox is designed to support and promote this process. But, how do you safely detox your liver? There are a growing number of trendy headlines and quick-fix plans for liver detox cleanses and diets, but what's even more overwhelming is the confusion around how to do one of these safely.

Furthermore, it's not a detox diet or cleanse that you need it's a dietary reset that enhances and supports your body's own natural detoxification processes.

When it comes to the natural detoxification process, the ability of a person to detox varies significantly, depending on many factors from overall health to nutritional status. Supporting your body's natural individual processes can help it regulate its hormonal and fluid balance, provide energy to your cells to promote a higher functioning metabolism, and improve your overall brain function.

UNPLEASANT SIDE EFFECTS

The buildup of toxins in your body can lead to unpleasant feelings like bloating, sluggishness, and lack of motivation. This is likely exacerbated by a lack of nutrients needed to fuel your body's natural detoxification system. If you choose to do one of the trendy water, juice or smoothie cleanses, you may not be setting yourself up for success. These can result in muscle wasting and an increase in hunger and fatigue, as they are often lacking in important nutrients.

In order to naturally detoxify your liver, the body needs macronutrients like high quality protein and carbohydrates, plus micronutrients like vitamins, minerals, and phytonutrients from plant foods that provide targeted support. What side effects can you expect when you go through a liver detox cycle? Some people report a few unpleasant feelings like headaches, congestion, irritability, nausea, muscle or joint pain, or fatigue in the short-term. This is most likely due to your body withdrawing from things like processed foods, sugar, and caffeine that you may have been incorporating into your diet.

A successful liver detox will help you get past any unpleasant side effects early on and experience much more enjoyable benefits. A liver detox, cleanse, or flush is a program that claims to take out toxins in your body, help you lose weight, or improve your health. You want to do everything you can to take an active role in your health. But if you think you need a liver detox, you should know that there isn't much it can do for you.

Your liver is one of the largest organs in your body. It helps remove waste and handles various nutrients and medicines. Most people think cleanse will help their liver remove toxins after they drink too much alcohol or eat unhealthy foods. Some hope it will help their liver work better on a daily basis. Many believe it'll help treat liver disease. Like most detoxes, a liver cleanse has specific steps. It may tell you to fast or to drink only juices or other liquids for several days. You might need to eat a restricted diet or take herbal or dietary supplements. Some detoxes also urge you to buy a variety of products.

ARE LIVER DETOXES SAFE?

There are medical treatments for liver diseases. But nothing shows that detox programs or supplements can fix liver damage.

In fact, detoxes may harm your liver. Studies have found that liver injuries from herbal and dietary supplements are on the rise. Green tea extract, for example, can cause damage like that from hepatitis. And the coffee enemas involved in some regimens can lead to infections and electrolyte problems that might be deadly.

OTHER THINGS TO KNOW ABOUT THESE PROGRAMS AND PRODUCTS:

1. Some companies use ingredients that could be harmful. Others have made false claims about how well they treat serious diseases.

2. Unpasteurized juices can make you sick, especially if you're older or have a weakened immune system.

3. If you have kidney disease, a cleanse that includes large amounts of juice can make your illness worse.

4. If you have diabetes, be sure to check with your doctor before you start a diet that changes how you usually eat.

5. If you fast as part of a detox program, you may feel weak or faint, have headaches, or get dehydrated. If you have hepatitis B that has caused liver damage, fasting can make the damage worse.

DO LIVER CLEANSES HELP YOUR LIVER HEAL FROM ALCOHOL OR UNHEALTHY FOOD?

There isn't any scientific proof that cleanses remove toxins from your body or make you healthier. You may feel better on a detox diet simply because you aren't eating highly processed foods with solid fats and processed sugar. These foods are high in calories but low in nutrition. Detox diets can also cut out foods that you might be allergic or sensitive to, like dairy, gluten, eggs, or peanuts.

Doctors say liver detoxes aren't important for your health or how well your liver works. There's no proof that they help get rid of toxins after you've had too much unhealthy food or alcohol.

WAYS TO HELP YOUR LIVER AFTER DRINKING TOO MUCH ALCOHOL

There's a limit on how much alcohol your liver can handle at one time. It has to work harder when you drink too much. Over time, this can lead to inflammation, scarring, or cancer.

If you're going to drink alcohol, experts recommend no more than one drink a day for women and two for men. A drink is 12 ounces of beer, 5 ounces of wine, or one shot of liquor.

Your liver can heal minor damage from alcohol in days or weeks. More severe damage could take months to heal. And after a long time, it may be permanent. Give your liver a break by avoiding alcohol at least 2 days in a row each week.

DO LIVER CLEANSES PROTECT YOU FROM LIVER DISEASE?

Your overall health and your genes affect your liver. So do your diet, lifestyle, and environment. Liver detox programs don't treat damage or prevent disease.

WAYS TO PREVENT LIVER DISEASE

Lifestyle changes can help keep your liver healthy without detox programs. These steps can be especially important if you're at higher risk of liver disease because of something like heavy alcohol use or a family history of liver disease.

1. Limit the amount of alcohol you drink.

2. Eat a well-balanced diet every day. That's five to nine servings of fruits and vegetables, along with fiber from vegetables, nuts, seeds, and whole grains. Be sure to include protein for the enzymes that help your body detox naturally.

3. Keep a healthy weight.

4. Exercise every day if you can. Check with your doctor first if you haven't been active.

5. Cut down on risky behavior that can lead to viral hepatitis:

6. Avoid recreational drugs. If you do use them, don't share needles or straws to inject or snort them.

7. Don't share razors, toothbrushes, or other household items.

8.   Get tattoos only from a sterile shop.

9.   Don't have unprotected sex with people you don't know.

DO LIVER CLEANSES HELP YOU LOSE WEIGHT SAFELY?

A few studies have linked liver cleanses with weight or fat loss, but they've been low-quality or looked at only a small number of people. Other research has found that a detox program's low-calorie diet may lead to early weight loss, but people tend to regain the pounds as soon as they go back to their usual diet.

Ways to lose weight and help fatty liver

Some of the lifestyle changes that may protect against liver disease can also help you lose weight and get rid of inflammatory fat in your liver.

-Eat a healthy diet with plenty of water, fruits, and vegetables.

-Exercise regularly.

-Follow guidelines on alcohol use.

DO SUPPLEMENTS HELP YOUR LIVER?

Milk thistle is an herb that contains a compound called silybin. Some people claim that it helps your liver work better and can help treat liver disease. But just as there isn't enough evidence that liver detoxes work, there isn't enough to show that milk thistle or extracts make your liver healthier. Some studies say compounds from milk thistle have helped ease the symptoms of certain types of liver disease. But no research shows that it treats the disease itself. Turmeric, sometimes called "the golden spice," can give your body a boost and may help protect against liver injury. But there's not enough research to support using it regularly for prevention.

Dandelion has also been considered a natural remedy for various conditions. More study is needed to prove that it works. Remember that FDA rules about supplements aren't the same as for foods or medicines. There's no guarantee that that they work the way they say or that they're safe. If you think you might have any kind of problem with your liver or complications from a condition, talk to your doctor.

WAYS TO A HEALTHY LIVER

The best way to fight liver disease is to avoid it, if at all possible. Here are 13 tried and true ways to achieve liver wellness!

Maintain a healthy weight: If you're obese or even somewhat overweight, you're in danger of having a fatty liver that can lead to non-alcoholic fatty liver disease (NAFLD), one of the fastest growing forms of liver disease. Weight loss can play an important part in helping to reduce liver fat.

Eat a balanced diet: Avoid high calorie-meals, saturated fat, refined carbohydrates (such as white bread, white rice and regular pasta) and sugars. Don't eat raw or undercooked shellfish. For a well-adjusted diet, eat fiber, which you can obtain from fresh fruits, vegetables, whole grain breads, rice and cereals. Also eat meat (but limit the amount of red meat), dairy (low-fat milk and small amounts of cheese) and fats (the "good" fats that are monounsaturated and polyunsaturated such as vegetable oils, nuts, seeds, and fish). Hydration is essential, so drink a lot of water.

Exercise regularly: When you exercise consistently, it helps to burn triglycerides for fuel and can also reduce liver fat.

Avoid toxins: Toxins can injure liver cells. Limit direct contact with toxins from cleaning and aerosol products, insecticides, chemicals, and additives. When you do use aerosols, make sure the room is ventilated, and wear a mask. Don't smoke.

Use alcohol responsibly: Alcoholic beverages can create many health problems. They can damage or destroy liver cells and scar your liver. Talk to your doctor about what amount of alcohol is right for you. You may be advised to drink alcohol only in moderation or to quit completely.

Avoid the use of illicit drugs: In 2012, nearly 24 million Americans aged 12 or older were current illicit drug users, meaning they had used an illicit drug during the month prior to the survey interview. This estimate represents 9.2 percent of the population aged 12 or older. Illicit drugs include marijuana/hashish, cocaine (including crack), heroin, hallucinogens, inhalants, or prescription-type psychotherapeutics (pain relievers, tranquilizers, stimulants, and sedatives) used non-medically.

Avoid contaminated needles: Of course, dirty needles aren't only associated with intravenous drug use. You ought to follow up with a medical practitioner and seek testing following any type of skin penetration involving sharp instruments or needles. Unsafe injection practices, though rare, may occur in a hospital setting, and would need immediate follow-up. Also, use only clean needles for tattoos and body piercings.

Get medical care if you're exposed to blood: If for any reason you come into contact with someone else's blood, immediately follow up with your doctor. If you're very concerned, go to your nearest hospital's emergency room.

Don't share personal hygiene items: For example, razors, toothbrushes and nail clippers can carry microscopic levels of blood or other body fluids that may be contaminated.

Practice safe sex: Unprotected sex or sex with multiple partners increases your risk of hepatitis B and hepatitis C.

Wash your hands: Use soap and warm water immediately after using the bathroom, when you have changed a diaper, and before preparing or eating food.

Follow directions on all medications: When medicines are taken incorrectly by taking too much, the wrong type or by mixing medicines, your liver can be harmed. Never mix alcohol with other drugs and medications even if they're not taken at the same time. Tell your doctor about any over-the-counter medicines, supplements, and natural or herbal remedies that you use.

Get vaccinated: There are vaccines for hepatitis A and hepatitis B. Unfortunately, there's no vaccine against the hepatitis C virus.

FIVE SIGNS OF A SUCCESSFUL LIVER DETOX

How do you know that your body has gone through a natural liver detoxification process? Here are 5 signs that may indicate success. You have more energy. Removing the natural buildup of toxins from your body is bound to leave you feeling energized. In the early stages of the Body Revive Diet, you will remove many foods that may be weighing you down like processed foods, added sugar, salt, and caffeine slowly replacing them and reintroducing healthier foods that can support healthy energy levels.

1. You notice clearer skin. Toxins in the body, especially when in combination with stress, can lead to skin problems. Even adults struggle with difficult skin, sometimes complaining of acne, dryness, or oily and blotchy patches. Helping your body flush out extra toxins, like free radicals and heavy metals, may leave you enjoying clearer skin. One of the foundations of the Body Revive Diet is adequate hydration, which helps remove waste products and may support clearer skin.

2. You enjoy better digestion. Your digestive system has its own detoxification system that protects your gut from harmful toxins. You may experience more regular bowel

movements, and any bloating or nausea experienced before or in the early stages of the detoxification process should reside. The Body Revive Diet emphasizes many high-fiber foods, which are known to support a healthier and more regular digestive process.

3. You notice reduced inflammation. Joint and muscle pain are common indications of inflammation throughout the body. This can be exacerbated by the buildup of toxins in your tissues, so following a detox may help you to feel less inflamed. The Body Revive Diet is high in antioxidant-rich foods which have anti-inflammatory properties.

4. You have an improved mood. It goes without saying that when you're feeling better physically, your mental state also improves. Detoxification often helps people sleep better, which also clears toxins from the brain and supports a healthier mood. Getting rid of toxins makes you feel lighter and happier both physically and mentally.

5. A successful kidney and liver detox is something that your body is a pro at managing itself. However, you can support your innate processes by choosing healthier, minimally processed, antioxidant-rich foods and staying hydrated. The Body Revive Diet program is an excellent way to guide you step by step through supporting your body's own natural detoxification processes and optimizing your health.

FIVE WAY TO SUPPORT YOUR PRECIOUS LIVER

Every day, your three-pound liver saves your life. The second largest organ in your body (after the skin), your liver works tirelessly to keep you healthy performing a stunning array of tasks. This workhorse filters everything you eat and drink, helps usher toxins safely out of the body, regulates blood sugar levels, stores extra sugar in the form of glycogen, and converts extra carbohydrate and protein into forms that can be stored for later use. Your liver also produces the body's "liquid gold" bile which breaks down fats so they can be absorbed, and carries wastes out in the stool. Your liver even breaks down old or injured blood cells. It stores iron. It stores clotting molecules for the blood.

It's versatile, your liver. But it is not invulnerable. Even this remarkable organ can be excessively burdened by the onslaught of toxicants so common in everyday life chemicals, poor food, sweet snacks and sodas, excess alcohol, pollution and the constant stress we all face today. We are routinely exposed to over 84,000 chemicals (many untested for safety because they were grandfathered in by the Toxic Substances Act). Then there is our "obesogenic" food environment, which tempts us to eat high-fat, sugary, refined foods that seem to beckon from every television commercial, store, and restaurant, and place a significant burden on the liver's detoxification system. Finally, the liver is impacted by chronic stress, a feature of contemporary life which can lead to chronic high levels of cortisol, and contribute to fatty liver. According to the Mayo Clinic, nonalcoholic fatty liver disease is common in the United States, affecting an estimated 80 to 100 million people.

Liver rejuvenation supports better health in the body from cholesterol and hormone metabolism to detoxification, energy and even cognitive function.

HOW TO KNOW WHEN YOUR LIVER IS OVERTAXED

What are the early signs and symptoms of an overtaxed or stressed liver? Are there telltale warning signals that your liver could benefit from a little loving care and extra detox? Here are seven tips your liver may indeed need some attention.

Excessive Fatigue

Fatigue is a common complaint the world over, and is often experienced when the liver is under stress. The liver converts glucose into glycogen, a form of sugar that can be stored, and then later released as glucose when the body needs a burst of energy. By storing and supplying the body with glucose, the liver helps provide energy and combat fatigue. If the liver is stressed it may become less efficient at regulation of blood glucose. Fatigue and sugar cravings may pop up.

Hormone Imbalances and Premenstrual Syndrome

The liver detoxifies more than chemicals and pollutants. It also detoxifies our own hormones, including excess estrogen. Not surprisingly, when liver function is impaired, excess estrogen may not be adequately bound and excreted. Signs of excess estrogen in women can include PMS, fibrocystic breasts, moodiness, weight gain, menstrual disturbances, fibroids and more.

Belly Bloat and Excessive Gas

When the flow of bile is stagnant or slowed, the gut shifts towards a state of dysbiosis, where unfriendly flora dominate, and constipation is common. The toxins from pathogenic bacteria then block detoxification pathways in the liver as well. With the resulting imbalance of flora and dysbiosis, excessive gas and bloating may be experienced after eating.

High Levels of Heavy Metals

Human exposure to heavy metals has soared, due to an exponential increase of metals in industrial, agricultural, and technological applications. From coal burning power plants to plastics, textiles, electronics, wood preservation, and paper processing, metals are ubiquitous in everyday life. Heavy metals can cause DNA damage and contribute to a variety of human illnesses. When the liver's detoxification pathways are impaired, heavy metals can accumulate in the body. In particular, the liver's stores of glutathione, which safely and effectively binds to toxins and metals, can be depleted. A comprehensive tri-test that assesses urine, blood, and hair levels of mercury can give a realistic picture of an individual's mercury burden. Other tests can look at glutathione levels, and levels of other metals in hair.

Chemical sensitivities and allergies

When the liver is under stress, individuals may find themselves more reactive to chemical exposures, including gasoline, kerosene, natural gas, pesticides, solvents, new carpet, adhesives, glues, fabric softener, formaldehyde, cleaning agents, medications and more. Seasonal pollen allergies may worsen, and food sensitivities may increase. The liver is responsible for breaking down excess histamine, and if it is sluggish, histamine may build up in the body .In individuals with chronic cholestasis and impaired bile flow, blood levels of histamine have been found to be significantly greater than normal.

Poor Sleep

Nearly 60 million Americans are affected by the sleep disorders every year. Sleep problems run the gamut, taking too long to fall asleep (called sleep latency), waking up too early, fitful and poor sleep quality, frequent nocturnal awakening, or early morning awakening. The solutions range from sleeping medications to cognitive reframing techniques, relaxation tapes, meditation, sleep hygiene, and more. But one simple solution may be to improve liver function. Sleep disturbances have long been observed in chronic liver conditions, and one mechanism may be impaired hepatic melatonin metabolism. Melatonin is the "circadian rhythm" hormone the hormone our bodies naturally release as darkness falls, and which readies us for a good night's sleep.

HOW TO CLEANSE AND REJUVENATE YOUR LIVER

Your liver is the only visceral organ in your body that can actually regenerate itself. If even a mere quarter of your original liver is left, it can regenerate back to its full size. Your liver's capacity for repair is immense. It just needs a little extra care and attention. Here are some tips for improving your liver function.

Improve bile flow with bitter botanicals
Bitter botanicals have been used for hundreds of years as both medicine and as aperitifs. They promote proper drainage of the liver, kidneys, lymph, and help support intestinal health. First and foremost, they support healthy bile flow, which is critical for digestive function, and helps balance your gut flora, since bile acids are antimicrobial. Remember, toxins and their metabolites are eliminated from the liver into the bile, and out of the body via the stool.

The classic bitter botanicals are potent yet gentle. They include gentian, milk thistle, goldenrod, myrrh, and dandelion. Gentian is often called our most bitter bitter, offering digestive support and liver protection. Gentian has been shown to increase levels of our most potent endogenous antioxidant, glutathione. It also improves bile flow. Milk thistle (Silybum marianum) has a reputation as a potent liver protector, also with bitter properties. Its most active molecule, silymarin, has been shown to enhance glutathione levels in the liver and gut. Dandelion is widely known for its tonic function on the liver, gallbladder, and kidneys. Goldenrod helps the flow of bile. Myrrh is antimicrobial, and improves bile flow as well. Guggulsterones are the molecules in myrrh responsible for its cholesterol-lowering effect.

Support the Liver with Pure Phosphatidylcholine

Phosphatidylcholine (PC) makes up 90% of the phospholipids in bile. Increased intake of PC has been shown to enhance prevent liver stagnations and subsequent liver damage. Phosphatidylcholine also is essential for the health of the gut, and is a primary building block for the gut's protective mucus layer.

Support Glutathione Levels

Your liver's ability to transform toxic molecules into less toxic ones, and then help your body excrete them, depends on two phases of detoxification. Phase I liver detoxification utilizes specialized enzymes to help neutralize innumerable substances. Phase II detoxification goes even further, and neutralizes the byproducts of Phase I. Then the toxins are removed from the body. To detoxify, your liver relies on many enzymes and molecules, but the most important may be glutathione. Levels of glutathione are naturally higher in the liver than the rest of your body. However, low levels of glutathione have been found in chronic liver disease.

Mop up Toxins with a Comprehensive Blend of Binders

Many toxins are reabsorbed after excretion into the bile. In addition, endotoxins from unfriendly gut bacteria, as well as bacteria themselves, can actually move through an inflamed gut lining directly into the bloodstream. This is known as microbial translocation and is associated with immune activation and inflammation. This puts more stress on the liver. There is no universal binder that has an equal affinity for all toxins. However, a blend of natural molecules that effectively bind a wide array of toxins can help lessen the load on our bodies. Binders to consider include bentonite clay, activated charcoal, chitosan, and thiol-functionalized silica. Because each has a special affinity for certain types of toxins, a blend will offer broader protection.

Support the Gut with Soothing Natural Pre-Biotic Gums and Fibers

Because binders can be constipating, consider soothing supplements such as acacia gum, which serves as a prebiotic fiber, and aloe vera, which has long been used in traditional medicine to soothe inflamed tissues. These support the health of the intestinal lining, normal gut motility and the growth of friendly flora, all of which can help improve liver function.

The liver is a multitasking organ, working to keep your blood clean, metabolism functioning and digestion system strong. It's also responsible for filtering out the nutrients that are available in the foods you eat and spreading them throughout your body by way of your bloodstream, and then eliminating the toxic waste that's left behind from this process. In addition to these vital roles, the liver regulates blood supply by ensuring there's enough blood stored, allowing the blood to clot, and breaking down damaged blood cells so that they can be eliminated from the body through urine or stool.

Clearly, the liver plays an important role in our health, and when it doesn't function properly, we are at risk of experiencing symptoms like fatigue, weakness, and digestive issues. It's important to note that liver issues don't only occur in people who drink alcohol heavily. They can also affect people with a poor diet, those who are under high amounts of stress, anyone exposed to air pollution and environmental toxins, and people on prescription medications or antibiotics. And since that just about covers everyone walking the planet right now, it's also important to note that a good liver cleanse can help to get this hard-working organ back on track.

SYMPTOMS OF A MALFUNCTIONING LIVER

When your liver has too much to handle, it can begin to malfunction, so if you notice any of these common symptoms, your body may be telling you that it's time for a liver cleanse:

Bloating and Constipation: When your liver is overwhelmed with handling a poor diet, prescription medications or environmental toxins that enter the body, this impacts your digestion. Remember that your liver is like the body's digestive control center and when it's slowed down or damaged, you will notice digestive symptoms like bloating and constipation.

Fatigue: It is common for people with liver damage to experience fatigue. Research suggests that this occurs because of changes in neurotransmission within your brain. And when toxic substances build up in your blood due to a malfunctioning liver, you may also experience a number of cognitive issues like confusion and mood changes.

Dark urine and yellow skin: Jaundice, which causes a yellow discoloration of your skin and dark urine, occurs when you have abnormally high levels of bilirubin in your bloodstream, which may be a result of improperly functioning liver cells. When your liver can't metabolize your blood cells as they break down, this causes the buildup of bilirubin, which ultimately leads to jaundice.

Hormonal imbalances: Your liver is responsible for breaking down and removing excess hormones, helping to balance your hormones naturally. But when your liver isn't functioning properly, you can experience hormonal imbalances that lead to health issues like mood swings, high cholesterol, and irregular periods.

STEPS FOR LIVER CLEANSE

If you notice any of the symptoms of a damaged liver—or you've been exposed to some of the causes of liver malfunction, like medications, pollution, and environmental toxins—you may want to try this 6-step liver cleanse:

1. Remove toxic foods from your diet: Processed foods, sugary foods and drinks, fast foods, hydrogenated oils, excessive alcohol, refined grains, and chemically sprayed fruits and vegetables put a heavy toll on the liver and can damage liver function. As part of a liver cleanse, stick to healthy foods like organic leafy greens, fresh herbs, cruciferous vegetables, coconut oil, and apple cider vinegar.

2. Drink raw vegetable juice: Juicing with a variety of raw vegetables will help to ensure that you're getting all of the veggies you need to boost the health of your liver. Juicing vegetables also makes them easier to digest, taking stress off of the liver and making nutrients more readily available for absorption.

3. Eat high potassium foods: Potassium helps to cleanse the liver, so loading up on potassium-rich foods is key. Some of these foods include sweet potatoes, spinach, avocados, wild-caught salmon, bananas, and white beans.

4. Do a coffee enema: A coffee enema will aid

detoxification and help to relieve symptoms of liver malfunction like fatigue and constipation. To do a coffee enema, combine 2 tablespoons of organic ground coffee with 3 cups of filtered water and bring it to a boil. After letting it simmer for 15 minutes and allowing it to cool, strain your mixture with a cheesecloth and use it in your enema kit.

5. Take liver-cleansing supplements: Some of the best supplements for cleansing the liver include milk thistle, turmeric, and dandelion root. These supplements support healthy liver tissue, strengthen the cell walls in the liver, and promote detoxification.

6. Eat liver (or take beef liver tablets): Organic chicken or beef liver is full of important nutrients that will work to boost the health of your own liver. If you'd rather not consume the nutrient-rich food (it can definitely be an acquired taste), then try taking beef liver pills instead.

DETOXING KIDNEYS AND LIVER: GENERAL GUIDE

These include all processed foods, sugar, sodas, and any foods rich in saturated fats. You also should avoid animal products, though dairy is allowed in small amounts. Do not drink any alcohol and avoid or at least cut down your smoking. Kidney detox, in particular, will benefit from a few days of a low-protein diet. This means excluding eggs, fish, and poultry, as well as caffeinated drinks and seafood.

Drink a lot of water and detoxing cocktails.
You should drink 8 glasses of water per day by default. However, when detoxing kidneys and liver, this amount should go up to at least 10. Make sure a few of those are not plain water, but detoxing drinks, such as pomegranate and/or cranberry juice (for kidneys) and beet and/or carrot juice (for liver).

Switch to a detox diet.
Maintaining a special diet is essential for effective detoxification. During this program, your main food should be fresh fruits and vegetables. Consume more greens that any other products, and get more carbs from Paleo-friendly grains, like buckwheat and quinoa. Juices and smoothies are good, but they won't provide you with all necessary

nutrients and calories. Be careful not to go overboard with cutting down your proteins and make sure all foods you eat are well washed and cooked when appropriate.

Get extra help from supplements. Liver Support

Detoxing kidneys and liver goes beyond removing toxic foods so that the organs can cleanse naturally. You need to speed up this process and restore the health of your vitally important 'natural filters'. Supplements can help with that. Liver Support and Milk Thistle will help protect your liver and promote its natural healing from toxin damage. Kidney Support and Cranberry Concentrate will do the same for kidneys. Be sure to read the labels carefully and pick a combination of products that will benefit you most. Your personal health condition and history matter most in this choice, as well as your diet.

DETOXING KIDNEYS AND LIVER: FINAL TIPS

Do not forget that a detox program must be short, not more than 14 days. You should start with 7 and watch how your body reacts. If you develop any pain or other issues, be sure to consult a health care professional immediately.

In case it's your first ever detox, start with 1-2 days every 3 months. Eventually, you'll work up to a 14-day program in 6 months. It's best to go slow as sudden changes to your lifestyle can be dangerous, even if they are changes for the good.

CONCLUSION

Kidney cleansing programs can vary considerably, but they often involve restricted diets, consuming only water, smoothies, and teas for several days, and taking herbal supplements. Proponents claim that these programs detoxify the body and promote better kidney health. However, there is little scientific evidence to support these claims. Most people can keep their kidneys healthy by eating a healthful, balanced diet and drinking enough fluid. People wishing to try a kidney cleanse or detox program should speak with their doctor first, particularly if they have kidney problems or other health conditions.

When following a cleanse program, it is important for a person to make sure that they are getting enough calories and electrolytes to support their body's needs.

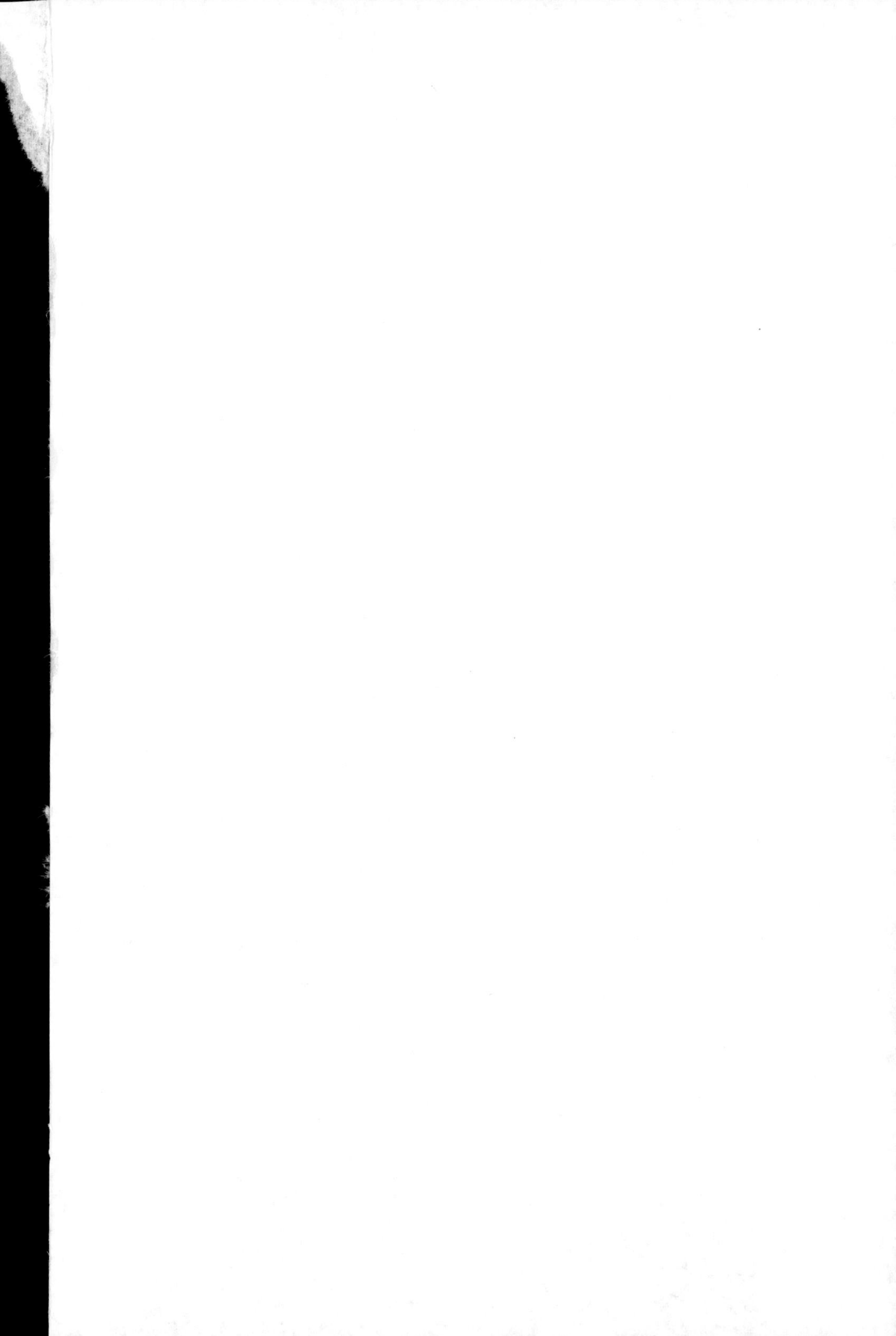